I0774395

BLOOD SUGAR REVOLUTION: MASTERING METABOLIC HEALTH FOR LIFELONG VITALITY

Unlock the Power of Balanced Blood Sugar and Holistic Wellness Strategies for Optimal Health and Longevity

Contents

Introduction

Glucose, generally called blood glucose, is an irreplaceable piece of our body's working, filling in as the fundamental wellspring of energy for our telephones. In this essential part, we dive into the focal pieces of glucose, significance to give a broad cognizance of its work in our prosperity and success.

What is Glucose?

At its middle, glucose suggests the centralization of glucose present in our flow framework. Glucose, got from the food assortments we eat, fills in as fuel for our phones, enabling them to finish different metabolic cycles central until the end of time. Keeping an ideal glucose level is huge for all around prosperity, as both high and low levels can horribly influence the body.

The Occupation of Glucose in Prosperity

Glucose expects a different part in our physiological cycles, impacting everything from energy creation to synthetic rule. Suitable glucose balance is basic for supporting energy levels, supporting mental ability, and progressing overall vitality. Regardless, when glucose levels become deregulated, it can provoke an extent of clinical issues, including diabetes, weight, and cardiovascular infection.

Why Changing Glucose is Critical

Achieving and staying aware of ideal glucose levels is imperative for achieving and staying aware of extraordinary prosperity. All through this book, we will examine the various components that influence glucose levels, as well as rational methods for propelling harmony and security. By understanding the meaning of glucose rule and executing assigned intercessions, peruses can open the phenomenal power of changed glucose in their lives.

In the subsequent segments, we will dive further into the science behind glucose rule, examine methodologies for assessing glucose levels, and provide huge guidance to building a lifestyle that maintains ideal glucose balance. Together, we will leave on an outing toward more conspicuous prosperity and vitality through the phenomenal power of changed glucose.

Section 1: The Science behind Glucose

In this section, we dive into the multifaceted systems that administer glucose guideline inside the human body. Understanding the fundamental science is significant for creating viable techniques to help ideal glucose equilibrium and by and large wellbeing.

The Science of Glucose Guideline

We start by investigating the multifaceted exchange between different organs and chemicals associated with keeping up with glucose homeostasis. From the pancreas' development of insulin and glucagon to the liver's part in glucose capacity and delivery, we unwind the complex natural cycles that guarantee stable glucose levels.

Glycemic File and Glycemic Burden

Then, we look at the ideas of glycemic record (GI) and glycemic load (GL), which give bits of knowledge into what various food varieties mean for glucose levels. By understanding these measurements, peruses can go with informed dietary decisions to advance consistent glucose levels and forestall spikes and crashes.

Insulin and Glucagon: Chemicals of Glucose Control

Vital to glucose guideline are the chemicals insulin and glucagon, which work in show to keep up with glucose balance. We investigate the jobs of insulin in working with glucose take-up by cells and glucagon in invigorating glucose discharge from capacity locales, featuring their urgent jobs in keeping glucose levels inside a tight reach.

By acquiring a more profound comprehension of the science behind glucose guideline, peruses can enable themselves to settle on informed conclusions about diet, way of life, and by and large wellbeing. In the accompanying sections, we will expand upon this information to foster commonsense procedures for accomplishing and keeping up with ideal glucose balance.

Section 2: Surveying Your Glucose

In this section, we center around the different strategies and devices accessible for evaluating glucose levels. Understanding how to screen and decipher these estimations is fundamental for acquiring knowledge into one's metabolic wellbeing and recognizing likely regions for development.

Instruments for Checking Glucose

We start by investigating the various gadgets and strategies used to gauge glucose levels, going from customary glucometers to persistent glucose screens (CGMs). Peruses will find out about the benefits and restrictions of every strategy, as well as how to utilize them successfully to follow their glucose changes after some time.

Figuring out Hemoglobin A1c

Hemoglobin A1c (HbA1c) fills in as a significant mark of long haul glucose control, giving a normal of blood glucose levels over the first a few months. We examine the meaning of HbA1c testing in surveying in general glycemic the board and overseeing diabetes risk, offering experiences into deciphering results and putting forth target objectives.

Perceiving Indications of Glucose Unevenness

Past mathematical estimations, we additionally investigate the signs and side effects that might demonstrate glucose dysregulation. From successive thirst and pee to weariness and emotional episodes, understanding these admonition signs can provoke people to look for additional assessment and carry out designated intercessions to reestablish harmony.

By becoming skilled at evaluating their glucose levels through a blend of checking instruments and side effect acknowledgment, perusers can make proactive strides towards streamlining their metabolic wellbeing. In the ensuing parts, we will dig into techniques for advancing glucose balance through dietary alterations, way of life changes, and designated mediations.

Part 3: Building a Decent Plate

In this part, we investigate the central standards of making dinners that advance stable glucose levels and backing by and large wellbeing and essentialness. By zeroing in on the creation and timing of our feasts, perusers can saddle the force of sustenance to improve metabolic capability and upgrade prosperity.

The Significance of Macronutrients

We start by examining the job of macronutrients — carbs, proteins, and fats — in molding glucose reactions and satiety levels. Perusers will figure out how to work out some kind of harmony between these fundamental supplements to advance supported energy discharge and limit postprandial glycemic variances.

Making Dinners for Stable Glucose

Expanding upon the standards of adjusted sustenance, we give viable direction on organizing dinners that focus on low-glycemic sugars, lean proteins, and sound fats. Through example feast plans and recipe thoughts, perusers will find how to make fulfilling and feeding dishes that advance glucose strength over the course of the day.

Ways to eat Out and In a hurry

Perceiving the difficulties of feasting away from home, we offer methodologies for pursuing careful decisions while eating out or exploring occupied plans. From checking menus for glucose agreeable choices to preparing with convenient tidbits, perusers will acquire trust in keeping up with their dietary objectives in different social and strategic settings.

By excelling at building a fair plate, perusers can enable themselves to assume command over their dietary decisions and streamline their metabolic wellbeing. In the ensuing parts, we will investigate extra way of life factors — like activity, stress the board, and rest — that synergize with nourishment to advance glucose equilibrium and by and large prosperity.

Section 4: The Job of Practice in Glucose Control

In this section, we dig into the significant effect that active work has on glucose guideline and by and large metabolic wellbeing. By understanding the systems fundamental activity prompted changes in glucose digestion, peruses can saddle the groundbreaking force of development to streamline their glucose control.

Exercise and Insulin Awareness

We start by investigating how ordinary active work upgrades insulin responsiveness, permitting cells to all the more successfully take-up glucose from the circulatory system. Peruses will find out about the helpful impacts of activity on muscle glucose take-up and usage, as well as its job in diminishing insulin obstruction — a vital driver of type 2 diabetes.

Picking the Right Exercises

From vigorous exercises like running and cycling to obstruction preparing and stop and go aerobic exercise (HIIT), we talk about the different cluster of activity modalities that can help glucose control. Per users will find how various sorts and powers of activity impact glucose digestion and insulin responsiveness, enabling them to fit their exercises to their singular requirements and inclinations.

Incorporating Development into Day to day existence

Perceiving the significance of normal development past organized practice meetings, we offer pragmatic ways to integrate active work into day to day schedules. Whether it's using the stairwell rather than the lift, taking a stroll after dinners, or participating in dynamic leisure activities, per users will figure out how little way of life changes can amount to critical enhancements in glucose the board.

By embracing exercise as a foundation of their glucose control technique, per users can open an abundance of advantages for their metabolic wellbeing and generally speaking prosperity. In the ensuing parts, we will investigate extra way of life factors — like pressure the executives, rest cleanliness, and wholesome methodologies — that synergize with active work to advance ideal glucose balance.

Part 5: Stress, Rest, and Glucose

In this part, we look at the many-sided associations between stress, rest, and glucose guideline, featuring the significant effect that way of life factors have on metabolic wellbeing. By understanding how stress and rest quality impact glucose levels, perusers can embrace comprehensive procedures to advance equilibrium and imperativeness.

The Effect of Weight on Glucose

We start by investigating the physiological reactions to stretch and their suggestions for glucose control. From the arrival of stress chemicals like cortisol to the enactment of the thoughtful sensory system, per users will acquire knowledge into how intense and persistent stressors can disturb glucose homeostasis and add to metabolic brokenness.

Focusing on Rest for Glucose Equilibrium

Then, we dig into the basic job that rest plays in directing glucose levels and metabolic capability. Perusers will find out about the bidirectional connection between rest quality and insulin responsiveness, as well as the adverse impacts of lack of sleep on glucose digestion and hunger guideline.

Stress The executives Strategies

Outfitted with the information on pressure's effect on glucose, we offer a tool compartment of stress the board procedures to assist per users with developing versatility and advance unwinding. From care reflection and profound breathing activities to moderate muscle unwinding and journaling, per users will find functional techniques for alleviating the impacts of weight on their metabolic wellbeing.

By tending to both pressure and rest as necessary parts of their glucose control procedure, per users can open the maximum capacity of comprehensive wellbeing. In the ensuing sections, we will investigate extra way of life factors — like wholesome mediations, work-out schedules, and care rehearses — that synergize to advance ideal glucose equilibrium and generally speaking essentialness.

Part 6: Enhancements and Glucose

In this part, we investigate the job of enhancements in supporting glucose balance and streamlining metabolic wellbeing. While a solid eating regimen and way of life structure the groundwork of glucose control, certain supplements and botanicals can offer extra help in directing glucose digestion and insulin responsiveness.

Supplements That Help Glucose Wellbeing

We start by talking about key nutrients and minerals that assume basic parts in glucose digestion and insulin activity. From chromium and magnesium to vitamin D and alpha-lipoid corrosive, per users will find out about the proof supporting the utilization of these supplements as assistants to dietary and way of life intercessions for glucose control.

Spices and Botanicals for Glucose Equilibrium

Then, we investigate the remedial capability of restorative spices and plant extricates in advancing glucose guideline. From cinnamon and fenugreek to barbering and harsh melon, per users will find the assorted cluster of plant-based intensifies that have exhibited viability in further developing insulin awareness and glycolic control.

Exploring the Universe of Enhancements

Perceiving the significance of informed supplementation, we give direction on choosing excellent items and improving measurements for maximal viability and security. Per users will figure out how to assess supplement marks, distinguish respectable brands, and coordinate enhancements into their general wellbeing routine in a dependable and proof based way.

By integrating designated supplements into their glucose control methodology, per users can supplement their dietary and way of life endeavors with extra help for ideal metabolic capability. In the resulting parts, we will investigate extra methodologies for advancing glucose equilibrium and by and large prosperity, coordinating experiences from sustenance, work out, stress the executives, and that's just the beginning.

Section 7: Past Glucose: Comprehensive Wellbeing

In this last section, we expand our viewpoint to envelop the interconnectedness of glucose guideline with generally speaking wellbeing and prosperity. By embracing a comprehensive way to deal with wellbeing, per users can develop imperativeness and strength that stretches out past simple glucose control.

The Association Between Glucose and In general Health

We start by investigating the extensive ramifications of glucose dysregulation on different parts of wellbeing, including cardiovascular wellbeing, cerebrum capability, and insusceptible capability. Perusers will acquire an appreciation for the interconnectedness of metabolic wellbeing with in general prosperity and personal satisfaction.

Tending to Fundamental Medical issue

Perceiving that glucose awkward nature frequently coincide with other ailments, we examine the significance of resolving basic metabolic and hormonal issues to advance thorough wellbeing. From insulin opposition and metabolic disorder to thyroid brokenness and adrenal weakness, perusers will find out about techniques for distinguishing and dealing with these interconnected wellbeing concerns.

Long haul Techniques for Wellbeing and Imperativeness

Equipped with a more profound comprehension of the multi-layered nature of wellbeing, we offer direction on growing long haul systems for advancing essentialness and strength. From developing solid way of life propensities and supporting steady connections to focusing on taking care of oneself and stress the board, perusers will find how to make a comprehensive system for economical prosperity.

By embracing the standards of comprehensive wellbeing, per users can rise above the restricted spotlight on glucose control to develop an existence of equilibrium, essentialness, and reason. As they leave on their excursion toward ideal wellbeing, they will be engaged to coordinate experiences from nourishment, work out, stress the executives, and other way of life variables to make a flourishing and strong starting point for deep rooted health.

End: Enabling Your Wellbeing Process

In this finishing up section, we think about the extraordinary force of adjusted glucose and all encompassing wellbeing rehearses in improving prosperity. All through this book, we've investigated the complexities of glucose guideline, dug into pragmatic techniques for advancing equilibrium, and embraced a comprehensive way to deal with wellbeing that envelops psyche, body, and soul.

Recap of Central issues

We start by summing up the critical bits of knowledge and focus points from every part, building up the significance of understanding glucose guideline, settling on informed dietary decisions, focusing on actual work and stress the executives, and embracing a comprehensive way to deal with wellbeing.

Resolving to Glucose Equilibrium

Outfitted with information and viable instruments, we urge perusers to focus on their excursion toward ideal glucose equilibrium and in general health. By putting forth clear objectives, remaining steady with solid propensities, and looking for help when required, perusers can enable themselves to assume command over their metabolic wellbeing and change their lives.

Pushing Ahead with Certainty

As perusers leave on their wellbeing process, we advise them that change is a progressive cycle, and misfortunes are a characteristic piece of the development interaction. By moving toward difficulties with versatility and diligence, perusers can defeat deterrents and keep advancing toward their wellbeing and health objectives.

All things considered, we offer thanks to perusers for their devotion to their wellbeing and prosperity. Whether they are simply starting their excursion or are prepared wellbeing aficionados, we trust that this book has given significant experiences, motivation, and functional direction to help them constantly. As they push ahead with certainty and assurance, we wish them achievement, imperativeness, and satisfaction on their way to ideal wellbeing.

www.ingramcontent.com/pod-product-compliance
Lightning Source LLC
Chambersburg PA
CBHW051900250726
48659CB00006B/2319